OVERCOMING MASTURBATION

Iyke Ihemere

themotivateworld.com

Catalog

INTRODUCTION: CASTING DOWN STRONGHOLDS

Strongholds are mental walls that become an addiction, attitude, or culture. It can be gotten from social influences, religious backgrounds, or demonic influences that determine or alter one's mindset and define the course of action of a person. Masturbation for you has become a stronghold, and that's why you have this book. This book will guide you step-by-step through how to debunk this stronghold and then help you build new habits to help you live an energized, motivated life full of passion and remarkable results.

CHAPTER 1: THE WHOLE ARMOUR

Life is spiritual, and the sooner you realize and accept this truth, the better for you. I'll leave the discourse of this truth and give you the bottom line, which happens to be good news. There are evils in this world that have a great influence on humans, but there is a name above all names that you can use to live a victorious life every day. The name is Jesus! The Son of the living God. Come to think of it, it's through the knowledge of that "name" (as a person) that I'm able to successfully create this book. So now, this book belongs to a class of gods (Psalm 82:6-from the Christian Bible), so if you belong to this class, happy are you. If you don't belong to this class or you aren't sure what it entails, you can either make up your mind now by giving your life to Jesus Christ, Son of the Living God, the one who helped me overcome masturbation and the one whose spirit has guided me to create this book for you. I believed in him and acted on my faith, and that was all the ritual needed to belong to this god-class. Today, I invite you to accept Him as your Lord and Savior so He can equip you to win forever! So do exactly as guided below if you aren't born again through faith in Christ. If you are, skip to Chapter Two.

UNDERSTANDING FAITH IN CHRIST - LICENSE TO WIN

Romans 10:8 NIV -- *But what does it say? "The word is near you; it is in your mouth and in your heart," that is, the message concerning faith that we proclaim:*

Romans 10:9 NIV -- *If you declare with your mouth, 'Jesus is Lord,' and believe in your heart that God raised him from the dead, you will be saved.*

Romans 10:10 NIV -- *For it is with your heart that you believe and are justified, and it is with your mouth that you profess your faith and are saved.*

PRAYER OF SALVATION

"Say this prayer below aloud and with faith in your heart, believing that God has heard you and that He has the power to spiritually translate you into His kingdom through your heartfelt sincere words."

Dear Heavenly Father, I thank you for your love-Son, Jesus Christ. I thank you that you sent him to die for me and that you raised him from the dead by your Holy Spirit. I believe He is alive today. I confess Jesus Christ as my personal Lord and Savior today. Through my faith being displayed now in His Word and in His Name, I have eternal life. I'm born again. Thank you, Lord, for saving my soul. I'm now a certified Son of God.

Congratulations!

Your First Christian Book: Now That You Are Born Again by Rev. Chris Oyakhilome

Chapter 2: CONSCIOUS CATALYSTS

There are activities that fuel the urge to masturbate. You must cut out these activities. This is the easy part. These activities include pornographic sites, magazines, books, podcasts, social media handles of shirtless men, butt shakers, and everything else that is SEXUALLY SUGGESTIVE both in words and action. This is your starting point because these materials keep your mind clothed in an environment of masturbation. Do away with that screen saver that shows an erotic body and replace that image with a list of things you want to achieve for yourself in the next 5 years.

Masturbation can make you lose interest in people and stop you from having meaningful relationships, especially with people of the opposite sex. When it starts getting out of control, it affects your dopamine receptors (happy and friendly hormones in the brain) and can turn you into a weirdo or a freak who is constantly in search of the so-called catalysts. These catalysts can be alcohol, cigarettes, marijuana, excessive eating, eating sugary things especially at night, and any other related drugs or habits.

This is not to say that the urge cannot come naturally, but when it becomes overpowering and causes you anxiety, it needs to be checked with the full lens of this book.

I particularly discourage the use of hard drugs like cigarettes, marijuana, cocaine, e.t.c. because cigarettes, as you know, ruin the lungs, make you weak, ruin your dentition and eye color, and can cause cancer and heart-related problems (making you start looking for a miracle – www.healingstreams.tv). Even though marijuana is thought to have medical benefits, it can make you forgetful, depressed, schizophrenic, quick to anger, careless, stubborn, and without feelings. Cocaine, on the other hand, can drive you absolutely insane and put you in jail, depending on the laws in your country. "Bar them out!" **"ALL OF THEM!"**

There is debate over whether alcohol or marijuana is bad for a Christian. The truth is that anything that has control over God's will for you and prevents you from serving or obeying God as you know you should, or anything that can induce you to say or do things you morally know are absurd, is bad for you, and you need to cut it off fast.

CHAPTER 3: SUB-CONSCIOUS CATALYSTS

Did you know there are sub-conscious habits that fuel the desire to masturbate?

Your eyes may be trained to look at the buttocks of every woman that passes by. Your hands may be trained to slide into your panties when you are about to sleep, and your social media handles may be positioned to show you things that lead you down that aisle. All of these and more have become sub-conscious catalysts, so you need to intentionally and consciously cut all the catalysts away, both the conscious and the sub-conscious.

There are friends that when you meet, you are sure you are going to do something bad. You are going to have to cut all of them off, and if they ask why you are avoiding them, tell them that you are recreating your world.

Proverbs 4:25 KJV -- *Let thine eyes look right on, and let thine eyelids look straight before thee.*

The Amplified classic of the same verse say:

Proverbs 4:25 AMPC -- *Let your eyes look right on [with fixed purpose], and let your gaze be be straight before you.*

As a sign of respect, you can choose to only look at people's heads and faces when they pass rather than their bodies. You can quickly and consciously retract your hand when it mistakenly or lustfully slides into your private area. You can consciously cut off associations both physically and virtually by unfollowing and blocking people who send or spam you with porn site links. By doing this, you are putting up walls against these triggers and diminishing the controlling power of masturbation.

What I've shared with you thus far are practical steps, and you won't be able to effectively attain the book's goal if you don't immediately put into practice everything I've shared with you, even though it means that you finish this little book in a week instead of an hour because of the instructive activities embedded herein.

Take a moment to unfollow all virtual catalysts, and if necessary, call the attention of your indispensable physical catalysts (bad friends and associates), informing them that you are no longer on their path and that you are now a practicing Christian. The Word of God says in **1 Corinthians 6:19** that your body is the temple of the Holy Spirit, who lives in you and whom you received from God immediately after you gave your life to Christ through the **Prayer of Salvation**. They will most likely laugh and retreat from you when you no longer engage with them on toxic levels. They will soon seek further explanation. Then you tell them about Jesus Christ, who is recreating your world and leading you through victory parades.

Also, not precisely knowing your purpose in life is called spiritual blindness. People rise to places of affluence and power and still find out there is something missing in their lives. If you don't let the active spirit of God guide you into fulfillment through the Word of God, it can either lead you to mediocrity marked by depressing repetitive tasks and cheap fun activities like masturbation to get by, or it can lead you to an exuberant life marked by lawlessness, lustfulness, sickness, carelessness, or selfish activities that never seem to find you real fulfillment, which is living like Christ on earth.

I recommend spiritual gluttony marked by continuous and relentless engagement and consumption of the Word of God, starting with the subjects that trouble you the most.

I go on youtube and search, for example, "How to deal with anger by Pastor Chris" or "How to deal with laziness by Pastor **xxxx**" and schedule to watch a series of videos on that topic or read books in this same light at times I would have otherwise used to have cheap or careless fun. You may notice that my suggestions are going in one direction. Yes, that is what it means to be a born-again Christian, but did you know that there are fake pastors out there? Some who look good but are working with dark magic and powers, and if you don't know how to discern the difference between a true and a fake pastor through the word of God or the gift of discernment, it's possible to get into a worse situation while looking for solutions out there, so stay with me because getting this book at this time is no coincidence!

CHAPTER 4: THE BIRDS THAT FLY OVER YOUR HEAD

There are catalysts which I call "the birds that fly over your head"
because you can really do anything to stop them.

Imagine entering a store or public square and the first thing you see is a
shirtless man or half-naked woman trying to get your attention on the
screen. This shows that we do not always have 100% control of
everything we hear or see, and this can be a tricky catalyst to
masturbation. So what do you do?

I want you to try to think of and write down something you can always
do whenever these birds that fly over your head get your attention.

____

____

____

CHAPTER 5: POWER OF YOUR MIND

◆ Are you a young girl who fantasizes about older men? See yourself as a morally upright GIRL, so you can begin to see that man as a FATHER FIGURE.

◆ Are you a man who fantasies about younger girls? See yourself as a morally upright FATHER, so you can begin to see that girl as your God-given DAUGHTER.

◆ Are you an older woman who fantasizes about young men? See yourself as a morally upright MOTHER, so you can begin to see that boy as your SON.

◆ Are you a young man or boy who fantasizes about older women? See yourself as a morally upright SON, so you can begin to see that woman as a MOTHER.

◆ Are you are both young? See yourselves as SIBLINGS.

◆ **DO YOU WANT TO KNOW A MORE EXCELLENT WAY? SEE YOURSELF AS JESUS CHRIST.**

Does that man, boy, woman, or girl look sexually provocative? SEE them as UNEDUCATED fellows. I use the word "see" because we are wielding the power of imagination to position our thoughts correctly. I also accurately used the word "uneducated" to refer to spiritual education.

If everyone was spiritually educated, then we would all know that our bodies are the temples of the Holy Spirit of God **(1 Corinthians 6:19)** and that we ought to always present them as a living sacrifice to God **(Romans 12:1)**.

Is that girl, man, woman, or boy a prostitute? See that fellow as an ABOMINATION to your mind so you don't become tempted. Avoid them as long as that would keep you save.

1 Corinthians 6:15 NLT -- *Don't you realise that your bodies are actually parts of Christ? Should a man take his body, which is part of Christ and join it to a prostitute? Never!*

The King James Version say -- God forbid instead of Never!

Did you know God is interested in your body and how you appear in public? In the Old Testament, they had a culture of wearing skirts (both male and female). In **Exodus 20:26**, the Lord told Moses -- *And do not approach my alter by going up steps. If you do, someone might look up under your clothing and see your nakedness.*

Do you sell your body for money or closure, it's time to repent and begin to see yourself through the eyes of the word of God. You should search for the "**Rhapsody of Realities—Daily Devotional by Pastor Chris Oyakhilome**" and begin to follow it diligently. This is important for all categories of readers.

If you gave your life to Christ recently or as a result of this book, then you should pause reading and go get the book—"<u>Now that you are born again</u>." It's free. Just enter the keyword on any search engine or search for a Christ Embassy Church near you, or contact me through my website or with information at the "LET'S RECAP" section at the end of this book. "Now that you are born again" is a small handbook or short pdf and a quick read. When you are done, you can come back and continue this book. If you are a veteran Christian who is struggling with masturbation, then continue reading.

CHAPTER 6: THE POWER OF CONFESSION

God, our own spirits, and demons can send us thoughts. Thoughts are " living things" because they are spiritually potent. Did you know that changing negative thoughts by seeing godly things, as highlighted in Chapter 5, does not always guarantee that the negative thought will go in the right direction and stay that way? Thoughts are as alive as spirits, and just as our Lord Jesus Christ commanded us to cast out devils or demons **(Mark 16:17)**, you are expected to cast out negative thoughts or suggestions that desire to reside in your spirit, because they are often inspired by these little devils.

How do you cast out devils or negative thoughts? You do so with words!

Out in the name of Jesus!

Go! Out!

Get out, you ugly one!

You defeated one, get out!

Get out, you little devil!

I declare peace in my body right now in the name of Jesus!

Philippians chapter 2 explain why this this possible in Christ Jesus!

Philippians 2:8, NASB -- *Being found in appearance as a man, He humbled Himself by becoming obedient to the point of death, even death on a cross.*

Philippians 2:9, NASB -- *For this reason also, God highly exalted Him, and bestowed on Him the name which is above every name,*

Philippians 2:10, NASB -- *so that at the name of Jesus EVERY KNEE WILL BOW, of those who are in heaven and on earth and under the earth, and that every tongue will confess that Jesus Christ is Lord, to the glory of God the Father.*

This is the reason why you can use the authority given to us "Christians" in the name of our Lord Jesus to deal with any and every situation including negative or demonic thoughts.

CHAPTER 7: MY JOURNEY THROUGH MASTURBATION

I got into the university as an innocent teenager. The only wrong I knew was to take cans of coca-cola drinks from home without permission. My father never wanted me to live off campus when I was about to start university because he saw the dangers of bad influences and wrong entanglements. I despised the school campus because it was extremely dirty, so I was rather glad I had the opportunity to stay off-campus.

My roommate from freshman year was a senior and also a chronic smoker. That year, I was always unsure about coming back to the room from school because the room was a like a chimney. All of that didn't move me to smoke because I didn't have any history or bond with my roommate or with smoking.

In my second year, I was amazed to find my secondary schoolmate in the institution, so I moved in with him. He happened to also be a smoker who stayed off-campus. This time, I definitely had that bond of history with him, and since I was no longer a stranger to the whole smoking thing, it didn't bother me so much that he smoked too. We did everything together, even getting food items for each semester. You know what they say about birds that flock together? They are usually of the same feather, and my feather soon changed.

It wasn't long till I had my first wrap. It changed me! Just like when Adam and Eve ate the fruit of the knowledge of good and evil. I became the lord of the chimneys and everything I hadn't done sexually before then was okay to do as long as I was "high". My roommate wasn't the masturbating type. In fact, he despised it and would rather hook up with real girls. I, on the other hand, a selective Christian at that time, knew the dangers of "joining my body to a prostitute and sinning against my body as it is written in 1 Corinthians 6:16-18."

1 Corinthians 6:16 KJV -- *What? know ye not that he which is joined to an harlot is one body? for two, saith he, shall be one flesh.*

1 Corinthians 6:17 KJV -- *But he that is joined unto the Lord is one spirit.*

1 Corinthians 6:18 KJV -- *Flee fornication. Every sin that a man doeth is without the body; but he that committeth fornication sinneth against his own body.*

So I said to myself, as a selective Christian, that I'd rather have sex with one girl all the time, so I wouldn't entangle my body with so many people. Before long, it was more than one girl, and each time I had intercourse with a girl, I felt guilty in my conscience and motioned to repent. So masturbation, coupled with pornography, became the all-time solution for what I call "degrading pleasure or cheap fun".

The Holy Spirit told me in my freshman year that if I had sex with anyone at that time, I wouldn't graduate in 5 years, which was the standard duration for a chemical engineering student, and guess what... You guessed right, but that's by the way.

It was okay to masturbate since it had low capital investment and low risk as compared to intercourse with a girl, so I enjoyed it for as long as I was high. It got to the stage where I didn't need to get high to have that burning desire to go another round. Seven years down the line, I began to notice that both smoking and masturbation made me lose ridiculous weight, and they couldn't give me six packs. I noticed that I withdrew socially and that my waistline and legs were getting thin with reduced stamina and weaker glutes.

Then I started looking for "fencers" and "keep-ups," i.e., ways to by-pass the ugly effects of smoking, pornography, and masturbation, but it was all futile and psycho. I went to church more often than everyone in my hostel while still struggling with all of this. To cut a long story short, I began to ask God to take away these habits even while at it.

I first ditched pornography and raised walls against catalysts, but then, the smoke was enough to fuel masturbation. I asked God to take away the smoke and he helped me in 2019 through his word to deal with it through the power of great personal sacrifice or offering, the type the bible talks about in **Psalm 126:6** -- *He that goeth forth and weepeth, bearing precious seed, shall doubtless come again with rejoicing, bringing his sheaves with him.*

It worked but even at this point, I didn't need the smoke to fuel the desire to masturbate. It became my sleeping and relaxation pill, but I noticed I was less productive almost every single day. This was where the real battle began, because at this point, I knew it was no longer physical, so I sincerely burdened God with innumerable versions of requests to help me deal with this challenge, and even though I tried doing different things to bind my hands and control my body, I noticed there was an evil spirit behind it.

Did you know you could listen to a "well-dressed" murderer and be immediately inspired to hurt someone as a result? That's the power of thoughts and little devils can keep inspiring you through things and scenes that seem harmless.

HOW DID I WIN?

I never stopped praying, learning and practicing "faith" and "authority" through the Word of God. Bottomline, I'm free thanks to God and particularly, the book "POWER OF YOUR MIND BY PASTOR CHRIS OYAKHILOME". I had read this book before, but I wasn't in the business of reading it over and over again until I became a Bible study class teacher and a self induced evangelist. After reading the book a number of times for the purpose of teaching it to others, Joshua 1:8 happened to me.

Joshua 1:8 NIV says -- *Keep this Book of the Law always on your lips; meditate on it day and night, so that you may be careful to do everything written in it. Then you will be prosperous and successful.*

I'm not telling you to become a Bible study teacher or an evangelist to stop masturbating, but I have shown you how I got over my addiction.

CHAPTER 8: DWELL ON THESE THINGS

Now, I believe that you are born again and have read the recommended book (Now that you are Born Again) and that you are learning to grow in your faith through the Word of God and prayer, there may be pressure from your immediate surroundings to reject your new way of life. You may discover that you are alone on some days when you would normally be chatting, dancing, or feasting with friends, colleagues, or even family; there is something you must do. Pray fervently to God for the kind of company that commands peace and inspires you to grow steadily in Christ. Pastor Firminus Kendra is one of those friends whose words, passion, and smile stick closer than those of a thousand men. One good friend is better than a thousand followers.

Pick up new habits like taking a walk at specific hours of the day to enjoy the beauty of God's creation. Be on the lookout for opportunities to assist and bless others with the gifts and blessings that God has bestowed upon you. Keep a clean and healthy life and diet. Get rid of songs and movies that inspire depression, wantonness, drunkeness, pride, anger, hate, racial discrimination, sex, and lust.

Phillipians 4:8 say -- *Finally, brethren, whatsoever things are true, whatsoever things are honest, whatsoever things are just, whatsoever things are pure, whatsoever things are lovely, whatsoever things are of good report; if there be any virtue, and if there be any praise, think on these things.*

Movies and songs are spiritual because they can use the power of imagination and confession, as discussed in Chapters 5 and 6, to subconsciously program your energy and way of life. When you get to watch or sing along to songs with degrading lyrics, you begin to act like those lyrics, and you could attract demons with those songs or through bad impressions gotten from them. I'm a script writer, and I'm working on good movies for us, and you can visit kingsview.tv in this regard, although this isn't free.

I intentionally left this point for the last chapter because people are usually protective about their music lifestyle and playlist, but the truth must be told. I'll help you if you are willing.

Typically, elderly people in nursing homes dislike being told to take drugs or perform certain exercises, even if it is for their benefit, because they have grown to know and live a lifestyle that has become natural to them. The secret to helping them imbibe new habits is to find a way to make the new habit or task their personal decision. So you have to cut off ungodly songs, but this can be your decision. I want to believe that someday all the songs on your playlist will be spiritually edifying.

I'M CHALLENGING YOU

◆ Based on the information shared in this book, delete 10–80% of the songs that have unwholesome lyrics and vibes that inspire depression, wantonness, drunkeness, pride, anger, hate, racial discrimination, sex, and lust.

◆ Go to blwsongs.net and listen to five different songs before downloading at least two of them that you enjoyed. Trust me, you'll like the songs. Add them to your existing playlist and shuffle your playlist for the next week.

Three times a week, download one new song from blwsongs.net and match it with one song from your old arsenal. Create a new playlist for the two songs and listen to them first on repeat and then interchangeably for a while, and whichever song blesses you the most, keep that song and delete the other. This is the hard part, but you I believe you are ready!

LET'S RECAP

1. Get born again if you aren't.

2. Put the catalysts under check.

3. Get and read the free book: Now that you are born again.

4. Cut off all catalysts.

5. Get your mindset right.

6. Finally, get the book, "The Power of Your Mind by Pastor Chris Oyakhilome" and read it over and over every day until you've gained mastery of your body.

7. Find a Christ Embassy Church near you and grow your faith through God's word and the Rhapsody of Realities daily devotional, which is also free worldwide!

8. Contact me through our my website or email address therealhouseof8@gmail.com for testimonials or for help in getting either or all of the other books directly from me for free.

More Grace!